Invisible

Amy Anderson

Invisible
Copyright © 2017 by Amy Anderson
ISBN 978-1546946991
Printed by CreateSpace, Charleston, SC
www.CreateSpace.com/7201839

For permission requests, write to
contactamyanderson@gmail.com

Cover by Whitney Robbins

Visit author webpage at
http://shadowlineswriting.tumblr.com/

For my family, who never told me what I couldn't do.

FOREWORD

"Raise your arms over your head. Okay, lower them. Raise yourself up on your toes." The doctor frowned. "Raise yourself on your toes again."

I complied and wondered how much longer this was going to take. I'd just started my sophomore year of high school and was in the midst of getting my sports physical for school. My mother (who was very patient that day) and I (who was not) spent two hours in a crowded gymnasium with hundreds of other students who were getting their own physicals. We moved through a slow line from station to station and waited for doctors to check our eyes, hearing, height, and weight. I thought the whole thing was a waste of time considering the only sport I wanted to play was golf.

The very last station of the sports physical involved the student and his or her parent(s) meeting with a doctor alone to finish up the examination. I thought the doctor they sent me to was nice enough, but I felt a trickle of irritation the fourth time he had me raise myself on my toes. At that point I just wanted to escape the crowded school and go home to enjoy some dinner and air conditioning. I was sure Mom felt the same, but she did a great job of hiding her feelings as the doctor knelt down and said, "Again, please."

I raised myself a fifth time. The doctor watched my feet, then nodded and stood up. He turned to Mom and rattled off a string of medical jargon that I couldn't hope to follow. Mom paid attention and accepted the papers with his notes. The doctor told us that when I raised myself on my toes, there was a tiny bone that tried to poke out the side of each foot a little. The doctor had me perform the exercise two more times so he could show us what he'd discovered. I was fascinated because I'd never even noticed it before, but there it was, a small bump on the outsides of my feet whenever I raised myself up. "Best case scenario, it'll be fine with a little physical therapy," he assured us. "However, it may need some corrective surgery. I wouldn't worry. The orthopedic surgeon I'm sending you to is the best."

We left that day tired and hot but relatively unconcerned about my feet. Surgery? Yeah, right. I was fifteen, and I'd never so much as broken a bone. My younger sister, who'd made five trips to the emergency room before she was five years old, was the most active person in the family. I was sure that if anyone was going to need surgery at some point, she would be the one. But Mom dutifully called the orthopedic doctor and learned that she wouldn't be able to see us for a few months. We scheduled the consultation, and then I forgot all about the whole thing until the day of the appointment.

The doctor who gave me my sports physical wasn't wrong—the orthopedic doctor I saw really was the best. She clearly knew what she was talking about and after our appointment she announced that I had tarsal coalition and pronation, which meant some of the bones in my feet weren't fused properly. And yes, corrective surgery (bilateral calcaneal osteotomies) was the answer. We could either let the problem go uncorrected, and then I'd have to have extensive surgery when I reached my forties or fifties, or we could go ahead and get it done while I was still a teenager. Naturally we opted to do the surgery that summer, and we figured we may as well do both feet at once so we could get things out of the way. The surgery was scheduled for June 6, 2007, just over a week after I would finish my sophomore year.

I was actually kind of excited. Aside from getting my learner's permit, the surgery was the most exciting thing to ever happen to me at the time. I'd never gone under anesthesia and I'd never stayed in a hospital, so the whole endeavor promised to be a thrilling new adventure.

It wasn't, of course. There was no way I could prepare for the amount of pain I'd feel after I woke up and both my feet were in casts. I had no idea how long a day could seem when walking was no longer an option. I wasn't prepared for the long, hot summer of sweltering bandages and the itchiness of healing. My family got me through it, but when the casts came off a little over three months later, to say I was elated would be an understatement.

We were told my pain would lessen over the next six months. I'd see a physical therapist for five or six weeks, and that would help me get range of motion back in my feet and ankles. It's hard to imagine how long it will take your body to heal following surgery. I remember thinking that if I could just get through physical therapy, then everything would be like it was before. I could ride my bike with my sisters, play golf, and keep up with everyone in P.E. class. It would be like the surgery never happened.

But physical therapy was absolute hell—I cried the first few times the physical therapist massaged the scar tissue on my feet. He was a nice guy, but I'm pretty sure he thought I was kind of a wimp. I vowed not to cry at any more appointments, but that didn't stop me from crying as soon as we got home. When physical therapy was over and I was given a clean bill of health, the pain in my feet didn't disappear. It got worse.

By the time I finished my junior year (12 months after my original surgery) we knew something was wrong. Mom took me back to the orthopedic surgeon and after an extensive checkup, she diagnosed me with Complex Regional Pain Syndrome. Of course we had no idea what that was, and when the doctor looked at my mom, I remember her saying, "If you're going to Google it, make sure you have a glass of wine in your hand when you do." That alarmed me. What could possibly be so bad?

Turns out CRPS is that bad. Complex Regional Pain Syndrome is a pain condition currently regarded as one of the most painful conditions in the world. It rates an average of 42 out of 50 on the McGill Pain Index—childbirth ranks around 37 and non-terminal cancer is about 25.[i] At the time of my diagnosis, CRPS was uncommon in teenagers and primarily affected people in their forties or older. There wasn't a lot known about it because as far as diseases go, it's fairly young (the earliest mention is speculated to be a doctor's journal from the Civil War). Currently, CRPS is garnering a lot of attention because many soldiers came back from deployments with it and some doctors now specialize in CRPS. However, back in 2008, the doctor couldn't help us much because she did not have much experience with it.

She sent Mom and me to a pain doctor who also lacked experience with CRPS, but he thought we could treat it like standard nerve pain and go from there. He did his best and frankly he was awesome, but it wasn't enough. Over the course of the next four years I underwent nearly twenty procedures with fourteen doctors. Nothing helped. We were even unsuccessful at the Mayo Clinic. Eventually we tried ketamine infusions, which are incredibly successful in a large percentage of CRPS cases. However, the infusions were not helpful in my own situation, and that's when we finally accepted that I was going to have to learn to live with an invisible disability.[1] I was 20 years old.

The thing about CRPS is that it isn't an obvious disability. If you pass me in a restaurant, you will never know that I suffer from intense daily pain. There are scars on my feet from all the surgeries, of course, and there's some swelling on days when I walk more than usual. But unless you see me on bad pain days, when I have to use a cane and sometimes a wheelchair, you probably will not know there is anything physically wrong with me. My pain level is almost never the same on a day-to-day basis. Sometimes I can walk through Target without too much difficulty, and some days I can't even walk to my mailbox. On my *really* bad days I can't seem to get my feet to work

---

[1] Throughout this book I use "invisible disability" to describe situations and conditions, but I frequently use the term synonymously with "invisible illnesses" and "chronic conditions." I understand that those three situations can be completely different, but they are also often connected with one another. Please understand that while I generally refer to these situations as "invisible disabilities," I am not implying that you are disabled just because you have an invisible illness or a chronic condition.

at all.

Living with any disability is no easy feat, but it can be even more difficult for those of us who are not visibly disabled. I've endured complaints and scolding from strangers when I use a handicapped parking space, I planned an entirely new career because my pain level was too high for my dream job, and I've had friends, boyfriends, and coworkers who claimed to be sympathetic toward my disability but let their actions prove otherwise. My disability is both visible and invisible since I sometimes use a wheelchair or cane, but I am here to tell you that it's the *invisible* aspect of my disability that is the most difficult to deal with.

Having an invisible disability changed my life because it forced me to look at the world differently. I suddenly became very aware of how frequently people judge others before obtaining the facts about their situation. I realized my relationships with my friends and family changed (some for the better, some for the worse) as a result of my disability. And I learned how difficult it is to handle living with a disability without a strong support system, along with healthy relationships.

Maybe you've had an invisible disability for years, or maybe you were recently diagnosed. Maybe you don't have an invisible disability at all, but you love someone who does and you're trying to understand what he or she goes through. This book is for all of you. By sharing some of my own experiences with an invisible disability, I hope to prove to you that living with an invisible disability can be difficult, but it is not impossible.

A DAY IN THE LIFE

I love the feeling of falling asleep. There's something so peaceful about laying your head down and settling into the comfort of a soft pillow and warm blankets. It is bliss.

I do *not* feel this way about waking up. When I wake, my first thought is usually, "No! I'm not ready!" I don't want to face the day. I rarely get a good night's sleep because even when I am unconscious, my body feels my pain. I've been told I toss and turn quite a bit. Even though I tend to think I can sleep through anything, my body has a different idea! When I first wake up I seldom feel rested. But after I accept that I absolutely must get out of bed, my next thoughts are on assessing my pain level.

Nearly anyone with chronic pain knows that some days are better than others. My pain level is determined by a multitude of factors: whether the day is sunny or rainy, how much walking I did the day before, how much quality sleep I was able to get, and how quickly I am able to put aside my pain and embrace joy instead. All of these thoughts race through my mind upon awakening—it is not generally a pleasant experience.

> **We are all star athletes running our own marathon. For some of us, the marathon is won by simply opening our eyes in the morning. ~Nausicaa Twila**

Getting dressed doesn't pose a physical problem, but

about 90% of my fashion choices are based on my shoes. The pain I feel is centered in my feet but extends into my ankles and lower legs, so I am restricted in my shoe options. It's not uncommon to see me in a nice work outfit...and tennis shoes. If it's snowing outside, my first thought isn't that I ought to wear a sweater. It's that I'll have to wear boots, so which clothes can I wear that will go with those boots? You'll probably never see me in sandals, and flip-flops aren't even an option. I'm sure people who don't know me think I have a bizarre fashion sense sometimes!

After I get dressed, I have to stand at the sink to brush my teeth. That's become much easier over the years, but when I was first diagnosed with CRPS, even standing long enough to brush my teeth was excruciating. I used to spit in a cup or bowl, and then my parents would wash it out. I couldn't even stand long enough to help wash dishes, much less take a shower. Even now, I take showers at night so I can go right to bed afterward because I know my feet will ache from standing for fifteen minutes. Daily hygiene takes a lot of effort!

When I'm ready to go to work I face my next challenge—going down the stairs. You may not realize this, but when you go *up*stairs, you don't move your foot or ankle much. You press down with your leg, but that's about all the effort required. Going *down*stairs is different. You bend your ankle and change the angle of your foot to meet each stair, then catch your weight as you move down. I can go up stairs without much

> **My health may fail, and my spirit may grow weak, but God remains the strength of my heart; He is mine forever.**
> **~Psalm 73:26, NLV**

difficulty. Going down stairs is tough.

These are all things I have to think about before my work day even begins, but I've been blessed because I know my situation could be so much worse. There are recorded cases of people with CRPS so bad that even a strong breeze against their skin is enough to elevate their pain for the rest of the day. I have to sleep in sheets made of certain fabrics and wear specific kinds of socks, but I know people who cannot wear socks at all because the cloth is so painful to them. My friend Alicia has CRPS in her hands, and her life is incredibly difficult. She has to use special dish soap because she can't submerge her hands in warm water. Showering is nearly impossible, and she'll never be able to perform activities like knitting or gardening that require constant use of her hands. Sherri has to be careful when she plays with her grandkids because they aren't old enough to understand why their grandmother can't push them on the swing set. Even though I am conscious of my disability throughout each day, I cannot imagine the difficulty some people face on a daily basis. Can you?

The difficulty goes beyond mundane activities, however. I live in Colorado, which is home to one of the most physically active populations in the United States. All of my friends like to go bike riding, hiking, running, tubing, kayaking, or even just walking in the evening. In the winter they like to ski, snowboard, sled, and ride snowmobiles. The options for physical activity in Colorado are extensive! Even though I have a great circle of friends who are very accommodating when they spend time with me, I am still reminded daily of all the things I *can't* do. I've trained myself to think positively and remember

> We live in a time when everyone's goal is to be perpetually healthy and constantly happy, and if any one of us fails to live up to the standards that are advertised as normative, we are labeled as a problem to be solved.
> ~Eugene Peterson

everything that I *can* do, but that doesn't mean I don't get jealous when I see people out for a jog. Every day, people with disabilities are reminded of areas of our lives in which activities are restricted. It's not anyone's fault, and we certainly aren't begrudging anyone their health. But disabilities have a way of taking over all areas of someone's life—even tasks as simple as getting ready in the morning.

I know I'm not the only one who deals with these

frustrations! Millions of people have invisible disabilities, which I wouldn't wish on anyone, but I take comfort knowing there are people out there who can relate to what I'm going through. In fact, both visible and invisible disabilities are receiving more and more attention recently because so many people have them now. Did you know that according to the World Health Organization, people with disabilities are actually the world's largest minority? Around 15% of the world's population lives with a disability.ii Disabilities are so common that you could see a person with an invisible disability every single day. Wow!

The Americans with Disabilities Act of 1990 (ADA) defines a person with a disability as someone who, "Has a physical or mental impairment that substantially limits one or more major life activities; has a record of such an impairment; or is regarded as having such an impairment."iii Later, the ADA mentions that a person is considered to have a disability if "he or she has difficulty performing certain functions (seeing, hearing, talking, walking, climbing stairs, lifting, and carrying), or has difficulty performing activities of daily living."iv Sound familiar? Can you relate? Do you know someone who can?

> **Strength does not come from physical capacity. It comes from an indomitable will. ~Gandhi**

Invisible Disability defines invisible disabilities as "both mental and physical conditions that are not immediately noticeable by an observer."[v] This may surprise you: of the 15% of the world's population that has a disability, a shockingly large majority actually suffer from invisible disabilities—96% of them, in fact![vi] That means *almost every person* with a disability actually has an *invisible* disability.

I want you to realize that if you have an invisible disability, you are not alone. If you don't have an invisible disability, you know someone who does whether you realize it or not. The numbers are staggering, but they don't lie. There are millions of us who struggle to get through mundane tasks like making our beds and going up and down stairs. It goes further than that, though. Having an invisible disability likely affects every area of our lives. It influences our relationships, our jobs, and our attitudes. I'll discuss all three in the coming chapters, but the difficulty within each area of our lives stems from one serious problem: people judge others based on what they *see* before they get all the facts.

THE PRICE OF JUDGEMENT

It's incredible to think there are so many people in the world suffering from medical conditions you can't necessarily see with your own eyes. One of the most difficult aspects of having an invisible disability is how frequently people make a judgment before they get their facts right. Has that ever happened to you? Or have you ever judged someone based on his or her appearance instead of learning the real story? Both?

The Invisible Disabilities Association says, "People often judge others by what they *see* and often conclude a person can or cannot do something by the way they *look*. This can be equally frustrating for those who may appear *unable*, but are perfectly capable, as well as those who appear *able*, but are not."[vii] Remember: people with disabilities number in the millions! The Invisible Disabilities Association goes on to say, "Most people do not realize a person can have hindrances on the inside that may not be visible on the outside. Their restrictions may not be conspicuous at a glance, but their pain, limitations, and inability to function normally can be debilitating."[viii]

First impressions of people are frequently wrong. How can we possibly understand what someone is going through if we haven't gone through it ourselves? Why do we look at someone and form an opinion without knowing what it's like to spend a day in his or her life? It's easy to feel pity when we see someone using crutches or a person who carries oxygen with them to the grocery. We can *see* that something is wrong because there is a physical presence of a disability and/or illness in that person's life. But what about the disabilities we can't see?

Consider mental disabilities. People with mental disabilities have no such validation. Their disabilities are 100% invisible, which means people need to take

> **The greatest battles of life are fought daily in the silent chambers of the soul. ~David McKay**

them at their word when they say that something is wrong. It isn't always easy to trust someone on that level, but without that trust, people with mental disabilities are left feeling as though they are doubted and judged incorrectly—and they frequently are.

We have to break the stigma of judging based on what we see. God Himself said, "Do not judge others, and you will not be judged. For you will be treated as you treat others. The standard you use in judging is the standard by which you will be judged."[ix] Yikes! If that's not a clear warning against judging others, I don't know what is.

It's unfortunate, but we tend to think we have all the answers. We don't wait to get all the facts about someone else because we simply assume we are right and carry on with our lives. If we see a person who is overweight, we assume it's because that person eats poorly or doesn't exercise. If we see a man or woman who looks tired, we assume it's because they didn't get enough sleep the night before. It's the same with invisible disabilities. If we see someone use a handicapped space and he or she looks perfectly healthy, we assume that person does not deserve the parking spot.

I admit: when I was a kid, I would stare at people if I saw someone using a wheelchair. I wanted to know what was wrong. Like so many children, I wanted to know *why*. Why do some people wake up happy and some people wake up sad? Why can some people run marathons but other people can't get out of bed? Why can some people go years without ever catching a cold and other people remain sick year round? Humans are inherently curious beings and children even more so. To be honest, I don't see

> **Everything is not always as it seems…we live beneath the lamps of our judging.**
> **~Christopher Poindexter**

anything wrong with a healthy curiosity. We *should* be curious about one another, but not so we can form a judgment. We should be curious so that we can learn to help one another and support each other in times of need.

When I was in my late teens/early 20s I had to use

those electronic carts at Target and Wal-Mart so I could get through the stores. I received some pretty incredulous looks, and there was a lot of blatant staring! Only a handful of people actually said something rude to me, but the experience was still frustrating. I wanted to ask those people to look at the situation from my perspective—I was barely old enough to vote, yet I had to use assistance to go grocery shopping, which was embarrassing enough. Having everyone stare at me just made it worse.

I do not get frustrated when children stare, though. They have to *learn* to know better. It won't come naturally. The beauty of children is that their curiosity generally stems from a place of innocence. I love it when kids run up to me, look at my wheelchair, and ask, "What's wrong with you?" I love that they genuinely want to know. They

> **For I can do everything through Christ, who gives me strength.**
> **~Philippians 4:13, NLV**

don't want to compare my situation with their own. They don't want to tell me about the time they had nerve pain or knew someone who did. They don't want to know what's wrong with me so they can decide if they think I'm faking it or if I'm in the wheelchair just for attention. They're asking because they are faced with a situation they don't understand and they want answers. It is literally that simple for kids.

Adults, on the other hand, are not so simple. Family

members, friends, coworkers, and even total strangers can take a bad situation and make it worse when they judge someone with an invisible disability. Sometimes they don't even mean to do it—in fact, most of the time, they probably don't. But the way they treat people who are diagnosed with medical conditions can make all the difference in someone's life.

Here's a great example of misjudgment, though it does not revolve around a disability. You've probably heard Aesop's fable, "Slow but Sure." In this story, a hare challenges a tortoise to a race that he loses due to his own arrogance. The hare judged the tortoise based on how he looked—all he saw were the tortoise's thick legs, the heavy shell he carried, and his slow pace. What the hare didn't take the time to learn was that the tortoise was patient and determined. It's the traits the hare *didn't* see that ended up costing him the race.

> **There is no greater disability in society, than the inability to see a person as more.**
> **~Robert M. Hensel**

If you have a disability, then you probably know what it's like to be on the receiving end of some harsh judgments from people who know nothing about you. If you don't have a disability but know someone who does (remember, 96% of disabilities are invisible!), then I hope you'll start thinking more carefully about what you say—

and how you say it.

I believe that unless you either have a disability yourself or are in close contact with someone who does, it is impossible to try and understand what it's like to have one. My disability opened my own eyes. I was forced to learn to give people the benefit of the doubt because I needed them to give it to me. People want to relate to other people and when they are faced with an uncertain situation, they take the only approach they have—they try to sympathize and relate. That used to drive me crazy because I felt like every time someone asked me about CRPS, we ended up discussing the pain in their great-aunt's husband's cousin's roommate's pinkie toe. It's different now because I understand that they're just doing their best to handle the situation in their own way, and there's nothing wrong with that. The problem was with my attitude in receiving their stories. I quickly adjusted my perspective and by doing that, I was able to appreciate them rather than growing frustrated.

> **I wish people would stop, sit back, be silent, and take everything into account before ever jumping to a conclusion and feeling the need to judge.**
> **~Barbie Mozer**

The truth is that no two people in this world are exactly the same, and that's true of disabilities as well. Just because two people have arthritis doesn't mean they both feel arthritis in the same way. Pain is different for every individual. The first time I met someone else with CRPS, I was shocked because she had a much worse case than I do! Hers is full-body, while mine is only in my feet/ankles. For the first couple of years after I was diagnosed, my only understanding of CRPS came from my own experience, so of course it seemed awful. After I met the woman with full-body CRPS, however, I learned how much worse my situation could be. Even though we both have the same disease, hers can literally prevent her from moving for days at a time while mine only prevents me from walking normally. That was the moment I began to understand that every disability is unique to each individual.

> There are good days and there are bad days, there are messy moments in my life and there are miracles...And despite the challenges, I know I am blessed. ~Lisa Copen

Understanding that every disability is distinctive was a huge step forward in changing my mentality about not judging people because it forced me to accept that there were things about people I couldn't comprehend, even though I have a disability too. I'll tell you something that no one wants to admit: people don't like to be told they don't know something. I didn't like the idea that I could judge someone and be absolutely wrong, but of *course* I can judge people and be wrong. The only way to avoid that uncomfortable feeling is to simply stop judging them at all. It's not easy to change a mentality, but it has to be done. We have to be able to look at people and refrain from judging their situation unless we know what they go through every day. We need to listen with our ears instead of judging with our eyes!

COWORKERS AND PARKING LOTS

The concept of not judging people with disabilities seems to be really tough in the workplace, whether it's coming from an employer or coworkers. Alecia Santuzzi says, "Workers with invisible disabilities encounter unique challenges compared to workers with other concealable identities and even workers with visible disabilities. These challenges occur not only in the decisions of whether to disclose the invisible disability in the workplace, but also in the detection and acceptance of having a disability to disclose."[x] Ultimately, it is no one's choice but yours whether to disclose that you have a disability.

It's a tough one, because we don't necessarily *want* to keep our disabilities secret, but at the same time, we certainly live in a world in which people

> **Then Jesus said, "Come to Me, all of you who are weary and carry heavy burdens, and I will give you rest." ~Matthew 11:28, NLV**

with disabilities are either judged immediately and not hired at all or they can't even find the opportunity to try. "Unemployment among the persons with disabilities is as high as 80 percent in some countries. Often, employers assume that persons with disabilities are unable to work."[xi] That is a classic example of judging without getting all the facts first, but it gets worse. "Discriminatory practices continue to deny persons with disabilities, as well as workers who become disabled, access to work. Two-thirds of the unemployed respondents with disabilities said they would like to work but could not find jobs."[xii] In this day and age, it's tough enough for healthy people to find jobs. Imagine having an invisible disability and trying to find a job, only to be told companies will not hire you because you are disabled!

I earned a culinary arts degree in college and became a chef when I was younger. Many chefs work up to eighty hours or more each week when they are first starting out. Because of my CRPS, I had to file a 504 with my employer to say that I couldn't work more than six hours a day, that I needed to sit whenever I was doing food prep, and that I could only work five days a week. Imagine trying to prove yourself in a world in which you work less than half the amount of time your coworkers do! For the most part, everyone at work knew about my disability—but only a few of them accepted it. I was frequently told by the people I worked with that I should stop trying to get special treatment or just quit the job, since I was obviously unfit for the industry. It was hard to hear this, and I had to remind myself constantly that they just couldn't understand. The worst time came one day when a fellow manager told me that he was the only "real" manager since

I couldn't do as much as he did. I was stunned. Our job titles were exactly the same, and we had the same responsibilities. I calmed myself down before replying. I asked him if he understood that I had a disability, and that I was trying my best. He rolled his eyes and replied, "No, you aren't. Pain is mind over matter. If you just tried harder you wouldn't be like this." I worked out the rest of my shift without speaking to him, but his words stayed with me.

It's not always like this, though. I've been incredibly blessed to have bosses and coworkers who are supportive and understanding of my situation. I even have a coworker who made me star spinners for my wheelchair—which he's never seen me use, but he knows I have one and takes it on faith that I do use it. Talk about support!

The good news is that awareness of invisible disabilities continues to grow. Even in the last five years, there were giant efforts made to make "normal" people aware of our situations. We even have an International Day of Disabled Persons every December 3rd! I'm certainly not suggesting that you flaunt your disability around the workplace or use it to

> **Living with chronic illness often leaves us battered and bruised. Sometimes the best we can do is just hang in there. When we persevere, refusing to surrender our hope in Christ, we may be down—but never out. ~Judy Gann**

gain sympathy from your coworkers, but being straightforward and honest about your situation can be a major step to give your coworkers an understanding about invisible disabilities, especially since they're hearing about them anyway on the news and radio while awareness spreads. If you can give them specific examples of what you need or how they can help, it will go a long way to promote understanding between you. Here are three examples:

Kelsey, who has a coworker with a hearing disability, says, "If you're talking to that person and you really need their attention fully in that moment, then it's best to get rid of distractions. Pull them into your office and shut the door. Eliminate any background noise. If the task is important, it's helpful to follow up with them. Send them an email or write a note, making sure they understand what they need to do." What a great example of how someone can be sensitive and understanding about the needs of a coworker!

Rose's husband has a learning disability. She informed me, "It's helpful to know what type of learner someone is. If you're trying to teach them, you can adjust your technique based on the way they process information. You just need to be able to accommodate that." Great idea! Bethany said, "You need to be open and honest about understanding their disability so you can make your judgments based on facts instead of thinking you already know. Have patience, and ask questions. People are more willing to talk about it if you are more willing to ask them questions." She's right! If we give people the information they need, we will all judge each other a little less and listen a little more. I would *always* rather have someone ask me for clarification instead of speculating on my situation.

The rest of the world struggles to understand invisible disabilities, too, not just your coworkers. One area in which I see this misunderstanding come to life is with handicapped

> Sometimes we don't even care if they agree with us; we just want them to take a mental moment to slip inside our skin and look at our lives from the inside out. ~Lisa Copen

parking. I interviewed people with invisible disabilities *and* healthy people for this book, but I was stunned by how many healthy participants said they felt handicap parking was "a bit of a gray area." Some admitted that they'd park in a handicap space if they were waiting to pick someone up, or if they felt they could get in and out of a store in less than five minutes. I was also surprised by how many of them felt irritation when a seemingly healthy person had a handicap plate, but after I explored the issue, it began to make sense to me.

You see, if someone parks in a handicap space and

then walks into the store, does their shopping, and walks out, people who *don't* have a disability feel slighted—but it might be for a perfectly good reason. "Many people are very disturbed by the sight of a seemingly mobile person taking the space of someone who is truly in need of it. After all, we want to protect the rights of people for whom these spaces are reserved!"[xiii] Thanks for sticking up for us! But remember—just because people look perfectly healthy doesn't mean they are. Trisha, whose daughter is

> **Don't be afraid, for I am with you. Don't be discouraged, for I am your God. I will strengthen you and help you. I will hold you up with My victorious right hand.**
> **~Isaiah 41:10, NLV**

frequently scolded for using a handicapped parking space because she looks healthy, says, "Just because someone 'looks normal' doesn't mean they aren't dealing with an issue you can't see. If they're parked in a handicapped spot but there's no obvious reason why, trust their disabled plate is legitimate. Don't judge."

I'm no stranger to this problem. I've received remarks from people who question my right to use a space—and often, they aren't very nice about it. I try to explain my situation, but the truth is that they don't understand that, either, and the encounter generally leaves both of us frustrated. I once had a woman literally start yelling at me in the middle of a Wal-Mart parking lot. I tried to explain, but she never once stopped for breath, so eventually I just got in my car and drove away. I don't understand why it's so hard for people to assume that if someone has a handicap license plate, they have a right to use it. Otherwise, they wouldn't have it!

If you view handicap parking as a gray area, think again. Even if you're only using it for a few minutes, if you do not have a handicap license plate or placard (and a handicap person to use it), *it is illegal!* If you think along the lines of, "She's at home, but I just need to run in for one thing, so I'll park here. I'll be super quick!" then you need to think again. I don't care if there are ten handicap spaces and they're all vacant. If you don't have a disability, then you have no right to use that space, even if you're just delivering a package or going in to grab one thing. It's not there for you, so please, *please* be respectful and leave those places open for those who need them. Even if all the handicap spaces are empty, a lot can change in five minutes. Furthermore, if you're using a handicap placard but the handicap person is not with you, it is a crime punishable by a fine, and the handicap person may have the placard taken away permanently. If you're using a handicap parking space without a handicap placard, you can be ticketed and even arrested.

I wish I didn't have to use a handicap space, and I'm sure there are people out there with invisible disabilities who feel the same. I can tell you that if I'm having a good pain day, I won't use a handicap space if I can find a regular space close by. Realize that handicap spaces don't make someone's life easy. They aren't there for our convenience. They just make it possible for us to get through the day with less pain than we may have normally. When you stare at people who look perfectly healthy but park in a handicapped space, it's patronizing and embarrassing. People who need those spots may feel shame at using a parking spot that's there to help them run their errand.[xiv] If we consider the possibility that maybe people are using handicapped parking spaces because they really, truly need them, regardless of what those people may look like, we can make their lives that much easier with our silent support!

SEEING IS BELIEVING

"You think you can do these things but you just *can't*, Nemo!"

Those of us with disabilities probably flinched when we first saw this scene in *Finding Nemo*. I think the reason we cringed has less to do with the rocky father/son relationship unfolding (although that's a bummer, too) and more to do with the fact that at some point we've all been told what we *can't* do. We've all had people we care about say something upsetting to us. *How could they say that?* we think. *Don't they know how much that hurts me?*

The truth is that they probably don't realize how harmful their words can be! Those of us with disabilities easily grow defensive about our conditions, and we often feel misunderstood. We don't know why we can't make others understand what it's like to have our disabilities.

Christina, who has fibromyalgia, told me, "If I could make a 'normal' person

> **If you are struggling tonight I want you to know that you are not alone. You are loved and so very worthy of it. Take my hand. ~Ella Hicks**

understand one thing about my disability, it would be this: Please be patient with me. I don't want to be like this; it is exhausting and discouraging. Do not think that because I look okay, I am."

Feelings of isolation and loneliness are fairly common in people with disabilities. One of my friends suffers from lupus, and she said being sick "makes it harder to stay in contact with people...it's not like I try to let my disabilities affect my friendships; it's just a matter of not having enough energy left in the day to keep up with them sometimes. I would give anything to have a day where I feel like they do on an average day. It's not like I can just try harder and magically get better." When we feel no one understands our suffering, sometimes we feel like we have to make people in our lives comprehend what it's like to constantly be sick or in pain. We may think we need to justify our situations to those who don't share them. Patty, who suffers from Central Auditory Processing Disorder, says, "I've become an introvert. I feel like I need to explain my issues with others I meet, yet that labels me even before they get to know me." Patty isn't the only one who feels this way.

However, closing ourselves off to friends and family makes having an invisible disability even tougher, especially because we tend to bring this isolation on ourselves. We get tired of having to explain our situation, so we just stop trying. Anne, who has arthritis, says, "I have hardened myself to a point that I do love and care, but emotionally I need to stay tough so it doesn't hurt."

We keep our pain hidden, locked away in a dark corner of our hearts that no one can get to. We hide the key and pretend that it doesn't bother us not to share this aspect of our lives. Many people with invisible disabilities simply stop going out socially, choosing to avoid situations that we know will be uncomfortable for us. "Even responding to a routine greeting, like 'How are you?' can be challenging. Many people with hidden disabilities would (rather not tell) the truth…One thing about being disabled, either visibly or otherwise, is that it's a lonely business.

> Don't think for a second I don't see how brave you are when you climb out of bed in the mornings. I am so proud of you. I'm proud of your confidence, your poise, your grace, the ease with which you navigate the currents of existence. And I love you for all your creaking flaws and elegant perfection.
> ~Rishika Sangeeta

No one knows; and most people really don't want to know."[xv] There are many times in which I have to opt out of a social situation, not because I don't want to go, but because the CRPS won't allow me to hike with my friends, for example. Rather than explain the reasons I can't hike, I simply opt out of the event and join them next time they do something a little less physical. And whenever someone asks me how I am feeling, I have a mental debate before I respond.

Should I tell them the truth? Should I say that I'm feeling rundown and tired, and a little discouraged? If I tell them that, they may feel awkward or uncomfortable. They may think I'm just eager for attention. It's probably better to just give them a generic answer like "I'm fine" and then ask them how they are doing instead. Even something that should be as simple as answering a generic question can become tricky when you have an invisible disability.

Sarah, who suffers from extreme OCD, told me, "the idea that I was imperfect and that I would be letting everyone down by being imperfect was a tough feeling, so it was better to seem OK." Laura, who has chronic headaches and seizures, says, "My husband and I have been dealing with this since we were married. It's become such a huge part of our marriage that we really don't know what it would be like to be married and be normal. It determines what kind of movies we can watch and if we can hang out with our friends. My disability impacts the outcome of so many situations."

Ultimately, it comes down to trust and respect. If someone can not or will not attempt to understand what we are going through, we assume that person does not

> **The LORD is close to the brokenhearted; He rescues those whose spirits are crushed. ~Psalm 34:18, NLV**

respect us—or the fact that we have a disability—and we feel slighted. It's worse when people don't believe we have a disability at all, since so much of the time our disabilities are invisible. That's the toughest part for me. If I open up to people enough to tell them I have CRPS, I want them to believe me, but unfortunately there are many times when they don't. They don't realize that by *not* believing me when I

> **I had people saying, "It's all in your head." Do you honestly think I want to feel this way? ~Sonia Estrada**

say I have an invisible disability, they are showing me that they don't really trust me.

I don't generally volunteer information about my invisible disability unless the need arises, so most of the time I know people for quite a while before they ever find out I have CRPS. The problem is, by the time they find out, they think I'm "normal." When I tell them I have CRPS, they want proof. They've seen me walking and smiling for a while, so the news comes as quite a surprise. They don't understand how they couldn't have known, or they wonder why I didn't tell them before. Occasionally it gets to the point where I feel like I have to show them the scars and discoloration on my ankles so they can see a physical sign of my disability. I hate it when I have to do this. If someone asks me out of curiosity or a desire for clarification, then I absolutely don't mind talking about CRPS. As I said earlier: I would *always* prefer people to ask me about it instead of speculating about my situation. But if I feel like I have to talk about it just to give them more information so they will believe me, it's hurtful. It proves to me that they won't believe what I say without absolute, concrete proof. I want to tell them to give me the benefit of the doubt—to understand that I didn't choose this, but I *am* trying to live my life as best I can under the circumstances.

It's tough enough to know that someone doesn't understand what you are going through, but for anyone to distrust the fact that you are going through it at all just fuels the fire. I struggled with this for a long time because I had a "normal" life before I was diagnosed. When the doctor told me I had CRPS, all of my relationships shifted. Friends who were there before suddenly weren't, and our entire family dynamic was different. It wasn't anyone's fault, but having someone in the house with a disability changes everything. Attention is diverted and suddenly priority levels shift. Weekend plans change. Work schedules have to accommodate surgery schedules. And just like that, nothing is the same.

I wondered for a long time why it was so difficult for people to understand what I was going through, but I finally came to the understanding that someone who does not have an invisible disability simply cannot fathom what it is like to have one. I'm going to say that again, because I think it's really important: if there are people in your life who don't understand your disability, it's because they *can't.* They can try, of course, and it's great that they do! But it is literally not within their power to fully comprehend something they never experience personally. They can't spend a day in our shoes any more than we can spend a day in theirs.

It takes two people to have a relationship, and believe it or not, it takes both of those people to understand how to live peacefully with an invisible disability. Those of us who have them need to understand that our

> **She may never heal, but if she does, it will be because someone held her hand through her darkest of nights without looking away.**
> **~Nausicaa Twila**

loved ones cannot relate to what we are going through. We can't expect that our loved ones will understand what we experience, just as we can't understand what they experience. It goes both ways. Those of you who don't have an invisible disability but love people who do need to understand that they don't want you to fix them. *You are not expected to have a miracle cure.* But we do need your love and support as we get through each day! We especially need you to believe us when we tell you how we are feeling. A disability is *part* of a person, but it is not what *makes* a person. It does not define who we are; yet it does define how we can live our lives. And we can't do it without you!

We live in a world where seeing is believing, and the unfortunate truth is that many people *do* lie about how they are feeling. It's terrible, but true. The worst part about it is that we've become a society that naturally assumes *everyone* is lying instead of believing that truthful people are still out there. It won't be easy to undo generations of this backward thinking but it must be done, and a lot of that will come from understanding one another.

THE OTHER SIDE OF THE STORY

I'm going to tell you a big secret: people who love someone with an invisible disability suffer just as much as the chronically ill people do. Yeah, I know—you're wondering how that's even possible. "But Amy," you say, "they don't know what it's like to be sick every day. They have no idea how tough it is to get out of bed in the morning. If they aren't in constant pain, then how can you say they suffer just as much as we do?" Here's how—because it's *true*.

It may not be as much of a physical suffering, but people who love those with invisible disabilities go through a lot! Think about it. Is there someone in your life you love? A parent, spouse, or sibling? Best friend? Now imagine how you feel when that person has a bad cold. It's horrible to watch! Every time that person coughs you flinch, because there's nothing you can do to make the one you love feel better. But you know that with enough rest, plenty of fluid, and sometimes medicine, that person will get better. Even though you hate watching people you love feel sick, you take comfort in knowing that they'll feel

> **And we know that God causes everything to work together for the good of those who love God and are called according to His purpose for them.**
> **~Romans 8:28, NLV**

better soon.

This is exactly how loved ones feel about someone with an invisible disability, but they have to watch someone they love hurt and know that person is *not* going to get better in a few days. The feelings of helplessness and frustration you feel when loved ones are ill are the same feelings loved ones have for the disabled—but without the hope of knowing they will heal soon. In case you don't believe me, I interviewed the loved ones of people with invisible disabilities and here's what they said:

- Jean, who has two friends with autoimmune disorders: "It's terrifying, and frustrating…some days I just want to scream at the universe for making my friends go through so much pain and hurt and struggles because neither of them deserves a second of it."
- Brian, whose wife and three daughters all have invisible disabilities: "It is truly agonizing to feel so helpless."
- Melanie, whose best friend has Lyme disease: "She has become a victim in her own life. It has been super hard to watch her get beaten down by this for so long."
- Bethany, whose sisters have invisible disabilities: "I get really defensive when other people don't understand, and they think that they're just being lazy. As I get older, I realize that people aren't being insensitive on purpose; it's just the way people are."
- Barbie, whose young granddaughter has Polyarticular Juvenile Rheumatory Arthritis: "Emotionally, this can feel like a roller coaster ride. The fact that we don't know how she feels and she can't express her feelings

to us leave us feeling helpless…That helpless feeling is the hard part, because all of us would take this away and carry it for her in a second if we could."

- <u>Ian</u>, whose wife has seizures: "The worst is the feeling of helplessness—watching someone you love struggle, and not even really being able to comfort them, let alone help."

- <u>Kathy</u>, whose stepson has severe anxiety: "It is gut-wrenching and like having your heart pierced…You wish there was something you could do to 'fix' it. We have come to realize there is nothing we can do other than be there."

- <u>Ann</u>, whose daughter has chronic nerve pain: "We have to live with the emotional consequences of watching her hurt and not being able to protect her as parents are supposed to do."

- <u>Ian</u>, whose husband has rheumatoid arthritis: "The sufferer's frustration level can be overwhelming both for him and for me. The changes in physical abilities come at any time, sometimes permanently, sometimes temporarily, so he never knows if he has lost yet another activity he enjoys or if it is just a flare up."

- <u>Rocky</u>, whose daughter has OCD and a mood disorder: "When she was younger and the doctors were playing with her meds trying to find the right combination in order to help her, I was required to sign a waiver with each drug, accepting responsibility for whatever happened to her while on that drug. I prayed every single day asking God to guide me and prevent me from doing any harm to my daughter in the process of trying to help her."

- <u>Lisa</u>, whose daughter has fibromyalgia: "She has no desire to be sociable and tries to find ways to avoid having to join groups…for me, being the mother of a person with invisible disabilities is very frustrating. I know that when people see her they have no idea of the extent of her illness. I know that many people think she is just making up her illness, and it makes me angry to know that people think my daughter isn't sick because she doesn't look physically sick."

You see? Loved ones hurt, too! Watching us suffer makes them suffer, and we need to understand right now that if we have an invisible disability, it means someone close to us is hurting on our behalf. To this day, my dad blames himself that I have CRPS. Despite the fact that the

> **And more than anything else in the world, I admire the way you carry your pain; even the air around you stills, humbled by your bravery and your grace.**
> **~Nikita Gill**

chances of me developing CRPS were miniscule at best, and despite the fact that I really did need to have the original surgery, he still thinks if he hadn't allowed the surgery I would be fine. I don't know how to make him understand that this isn't the case, but seeing me hurt makes him hurt. It's the same for the rest of my family— once, when someone gave me a tough time about my disability, I had a brief moment in which I honestly thought my sister was going to clock that person in the face! The level of emotion that exists for anyone dealing with an invisible disability or loving someone who has one can be very high. My family is incredibly protective of me and we've learned to deal with my CRPS—but we learned to deal with it together.

However, it wasn't always this way. My family has always been very close, but there were certainly times of doubt when we were first learning to adjust to my new life. My siblings didn't quite understand what it was going to be like for me to live with a disability, and the truth was, I no longer understood what their lives were like, either, because there was so much I couldn't relate to anymore. The reason I'm telling you this is because those of us with invisible disabilities are just as much at fault for judging others as others are for judging us. Sarah, who I quoted earlier, says, "Having any disability creates a line between people. People don't know how to handle it. They don't understand. As much as I understand my disability (or don't, some days), I don't understand the next person's." If a person makes a comment doubting the existence of our disability, it's easy to get defensive by saying, "Well, you don't have it, so you don't understand." We aren't wrong, but we could definitely

> **"I am something new,"** you must tell yourself. **"I am the beginning and end of a story that will never be lived again. I am new earth and new air and new words...I am significant."**
> ~Christopher Poindexter

handle this better. Instead of bottling our feelings and allowing social isolation to become even more of a problem in our lives, we could try to explain the situation.

Melanie, who I quoted earlier and whose friend has Lyme disease, told me, "Although I know unseen disabilities can be very private, I wish more people would share their stories to spread awareness and garner support." See?

You might be surprised how receptive healthy people are to hearing about invisible disabilities. If a situation arises in which someone learns of an invisible disability and you share your experiences with that person, things could actually turn out just fine!

I know that talking about our disabilities can make us very sensitive, and this is sometimes toughest when people offer us advice. It can be pretty annoying when people constantly tell us what we should do to get better, even though we've probably tried most of their suggested cures already. "Get more sleep," or "take it easy," are some of the easiest pieces of advice to hear, but it's harder to take when they say things like, "Well, have you asked your doctor about this new procedure?" In my opinion, it gets *really* tricky when people act like they know all about your situation, when in fact they don't. I've reached the point in my life where I can thank them for their advice and move on, but it took me a while! People used to tell me, "CRPS? That's a pain thing, right? So if you just take some extra strength Tylenol or Aleve you should be fine. Problem solved!" Um…no.

When people offer advice on a subject that we deal with on a daily basis but they never experience, it can frequently come across as insulting. Lisa Copen said, "The scattered advice from people who knew nothing about my illness felt like a personal attack against my intellect." I feel the same way! As people come to me and tell me all the things I should do to take care of my "problem," I just want to ask, "What do you think I've been doing the last ten years?" I want to remind them that I've tried *dozens* of unsuccessful procedures and medications.

Sometimes when they offer this advice it isn't meant to be insulting. Perhaps they really are just trying to help. "Just don't think about the pain" and "you'll grow out of it" are my very favorite accidental insults. I also find humor in, "Maybe if you just tried a little harder you'd get better." When someone we love says something hurtful to us—insinuating that our condition is in our head, or that we aren't trying hard enough—that person actually might be trying to say something else. Maybe the loved one is trying to rationalize our condition in his or her own mind. If an individual feels sick, then that person can take care of their body and get better. Maybe others just don't understand

> **Everyone suffers on this earth, and no one gets through life without a few scars. We cannot demand sensitivity.**
> **~Lisa Copen**

that it's not like that for those of us with chronic conditions. If they say "You'll grow out of it," they could be verbalizing a hope they have for us: that one day, we will wake up feeling better than ever before. Just because we take something people say personally doesn't mean it was said with the intent to hurt us.

It's important to remember that we are not the only ones who go through a difficult time when we have an invisible disability. Our loved ones are just as affected as we are, even if they don't feel the physicality of the situation. If we can understand this, it'll be easier to listen with our ears instead of judging with our eyes.

ATTITUDE

It's so easy to feel discouraged when you deal with daily pain. In fact, finding joy can be one of the most difficult parts of your day. I hope you're now on your way to a new appreciation of your loved ones, and that will make a huge difference in your life. Not judging people will bring you more peace than you realize. However, a huge difference between people who *suffer* from disabilities and people who can *live* with them has a lot to do with their attitude.

It's always been my belief that joy is something you have to make an effort to grasp wholeheartedly. Certain events, people, places, and even things may make you happy. That's great! But I'm talking about *joy*, the kind of delight that grows in your very soul and spills into every area of your life. Happiness can last five minutes or even a week or two, but there is inevitably a moment in which one of a million other emotions will cover that happiness. Humans are emotional beings, after all. Remembering to be joyful

> **A bad attitude can literally block love, blessings, and destiny from finding you. Don't be the reason you don't succeed. ~Mandy Hale**

even when things seem their worst is something you have to *decide* to do. Eventually it'll become second nature, but it takes training.

First, you have to accept your situation. Either you must learn to live with a disability, or you learn to help someone you love who will have to adjust his or her life accordingly. Being diagnosed with an invisible disability is sometimes compared to a type of death because the life of the diagnosed person is going to change drastically. We have to say goodbye to the lives we lived before. Things will not be the same, and we cannot cling to the remnant of our healthy life. It's not accessible to us anymore.

> **Remember how far you've come, not just how far you have to go. You are not where you want to be, but neither are you where you used to be.**
> **~Rick Warren**

People diagnosed with chronic conditions are going to need time to grieve for what they've lost. There may be a period in which they are so frustrated, depressed, and upset that they can't even think about what it was like to be happy, much less that they will be happy again. Loved ones may feel this way, too. You all need to be able to grieve and move on, either together or separately (though I recommend together!). You're going to have to completely rebuild your life, which "can seem like a daunting task. Take heart. With a little knowledge, creativity, and encouragement from others, it's possible. Just remember that God has a plan and purpose for your life, and He will lead you each step of the way."[xvi]

It's easy to be bitter about the situation and question why God let this happen to you in the first place. Richard Leonard, a minister with a PhD in Biblical Studies, suggests a helpful route to take when

> **As we live each day with the memory of our old lives, we do not have to be sad or confused about who we are now. We can live with the losses and realize that if they propel us to Christ, then we have gained a great deal more than we have lost.**
> **~Christina Smith**

you fall into this pit. "Follow the example of the Psalmists," he says, "who sometimes cry out to God as though taking Him to task for their problems, but who persist in their conversation with Him; eventually [they received] an answer, reinforcing His faithfulness to His servants." You see, even through these difficult periods, God is still molding you. He has a plan! Just because we can't see the goal doesn't mean we aren't approaching it.

For those who don't have an invisible disability but love someone who does, it's important to remember that when someone is diagnosed with a chronic illness or defined as "disabled," this means his or her entire life is going to change. Everything about the daily routine they once knew may be affected, and it'll take a while for that person to get used to all the changes. Psychologists call this process "redefining normal." Mary Yerkes says, "Many with chronic illness have rebuilt their lives and have gone on to launch new ministries, careers, and friendships. Others have developed gifts and talents they never knew they had."[xvii] The most important thing you can do is continue to be supportive on your loved one's bad days, not just good days.

How can people possibly choose joy when they feel so much pain and unhappiness? Remember, it is a *choice*. The first step toward choosing joy is reconciling yourself to the fact that you have an invisible disability now, or someone you love does. It's okay to have bad days and to grieve for what you've lost, but make sure you keep bad days in perspective! Don't let your pain drag you down— wear it like armor, not chains. With every breath, inhale courage and exhale bitterness. You were never created to be unhappy, or ashamed, or depressed. You were created to shine! You've gotten through every single bad day in your life so far, and you will get through the rest.

One technique for experiencing joy that works well for me is praying as soon as I wake up. As I mentioned earlier, I don't initially feel happy when I wake up in the morning, which has nothing to do with the fact that it's morning. While I was sleeping, I was not conscious of my pain, but when I woke, it all came back to me again. The first few minutes of my day are the hardest. I frequently reference God's word in 2 Corinthians 12:9, when God promises us, "…My grace is all you need. My power works best in weakness" (NLV). God's promises are solid! The Bible is full of His assurances that He will never leave us, that He has a plan, and that He is in control. And if the God of all comfort promises that you'll be okay, then believe that you will be. Remember, God knows the limits of your endurance. Starting your day in prayer, even if you aren't out of bed yet (God understands!), will make it a lot easier to face the day. Not only does He hear you, but I find that praying when I wake up reminds me that God is there and ready to help me each day.

Listening to music throughout the day can also help you choose joy. There's a *lot* of music out there that reminds us of God's faithfulness, of the power of a smile, and of joy itself. I have a "pain playlist" that I tend to listen to on the way to work or as I'm eating breakfast. I included a few songs in the back of this book in case you need some joy songs in your life (and I believe that you do!). Music is a fantastic way to remind yourself to choose joy. My pain playlist is a mix of upbeat songs and slower songs, and I certainly don't listen to it *every* day. But if you're having a particularly bad minute and you need a quick reminder that joy is something you have

> **Growth is simply learning how to suffer gracefully, elegantly, and not letting your pain tear you apart.**
> **~Nikita Gill**

to seize all on your own, a song can be a wonderful solution.

Other than accepting your invisible disability, praying, and listening to music, how else can you keep joy in your life? This might be a tough one, but you need to eliminate

> **The flames cannot destroy your heart, for diamonds do not burn. ~Matt Eayre**

poisonous relationships from your life. If you have relationships that are not uplifting and healthy for all involved, it might be time to reconsider those relationships. Georgia Schaffer said, "Few things are more draining than dysfunctional relationships. People who consistently blame you for their problems, criticize your choices, and discount your feelings are toxic. If being in someone's company continually drains you, it might be a sign of an unhealthy relationship. Learn to establish healthy boundaries."[xviii]

It's not easy. I can tell you that letting go of someone whom you feel is bringing you down can be agonizing. But if there's someone in your life who causes you more frustration than happiness, more pain than healing, and makes you feel more drained than energized, you may need to reevaluate the relationship you have with that person. It's essential that you have a strong support system in all areas of your life. Family, friends, and coworkers are all people you will interact with on a semi-regular basis, so make sure the relationships you have with those people are positive and joyful! If you're struggling with this, there are some great resources listed in the back of this book that may help.

Now, those of you who do not have invisible disabilities may be wondering why so much of the responsibility with these relationships is on you. So your loved one is hurting—you have stuff going on in your life, too! And you're right; you need love and support just as much as he or she does. Here's the difference: if your loved one is diagnosed with a chronic condition, that is *it*. "Chronic" means "long-term," and a lot of the most common invisible disabilities don't have cures. While you may be worrying about paying your bills, your loved one may be worrying about getting out of bed each day. I'm not saying that the troubles in your life are any less significant,

> **"For I know the plans I have for you," says the Lord. "They are plans for good and not for disaster, to give you a future and a hope."**
> **~Jeremiah 29:11, NLV**

but I *am* saying that you, at least, have hope. You know that if you work hard, you'll make enough money to pay for your car. You know that if you make an effort, you can get through that project you've been working on. The people you love who have invisible disabilities don't necessarily have this hope. For them, it's not a matter of trying harder. It's a matter of trying at all.

My friend Amanda gave me some insight into caring for someone with an invisible disability. "Just love that person and try to help her out in whatever way possible. Be as understanding as possible and learn as much as you can about the disease so you can empathize with her." The more involved you are with someone's invisible disability, the more joyous your relationship can be. Chau, whose son has autism, actually feels his son's condition has been insightful for the whole family. "I think having a special needs child has taught us to slow down. We have appreciated every little development," he says. "There are many challenges, but there are also many small victories when the obstacles are vanquished."

I was blessed with a wonderful family, and I never feel more joyful than when I spend time with them. When we are together, I'm able to forget about my pain for a little while. I get to support them with their own lives, and at the same time, they make sure that I don't feel alone in my situation. The support of family and friends is vital to keeping joy in your life!

If people who have invisible disabilities can remember that they must choose happiness every morning when they wake up, and be as supportive to their loved ones as possible, their relationships will only improve. If those who love people with invisible disabilities can sympathize and try to understand the condition, it will be that much easier to bring joy to the relationship.

> **Be an encourager. The world has plenty of critics already. ~Dave Willis**

Developing joyous relationships is the first step to mutual understanding, and mutual understanding is a key element in comprehending invisible disabilities. You can do it!

Let's start listening with our ears instead of judging with our eyes—all of us.

AFTERWORD

If you have an invisible disability, I hope you understand how your situation affects those around you and how you and your loved ones can still live together with joy. If you love people who have invisible disabilities, I hope I shared a little of what their life may be like, and how you can help them even if you can't really understand what they go through.

I'd love to speak more with anyone who has questions or would like more information about invisible disabilities! You can reach me at contactamyanderson@gmail.com. I've included some resources in the back of this book for anyone who would like further reference, and I hope you take the opportunity to look through them. In the meantime, listen with your ears instead of judging with your eyes!

FURTHER RESOURCES

If you found this book helpful—and I sincerely hope you did!—here are a few more resources you can use in your own journey toward understanding invisible disabilities. I quoted from these sources several times throughout my book, so they may look familiar to you.

But You LOOK Good: How to Encourage and Understand People Living with Illness and Pain, by Wayne and Sherri Connell.

The God of All Comfort: Devotions of Hope for Those Who Chronically Suffer, by Judy Gann.

Why Can't I Make People Understand? Discovering the Validation Those with Chronic Illness Seek and Why, by Lisa Copen.

If you don't have the time to read the books listed above, you can also check out these websites:

https://invisibledisabilities.org
http://www.focusonthefamily.com
http://restministries.com
http://www.idpwd.com.au
https://powerofpain.org/

PAIN PLAYLIST

Music is proven to help improve mood, pain level, and energy. Personally, I find this especially true for those of us with chronic conditions! There are times when I listen to music to remind myself that the sun will continue to rise and God is always faithful. Here are a few of my favorites:

1. "Joy" by Newsboys
2. "Even If" by Kutless
3. "God is God" by Steven Curtis Chapman
4. "Speak Life" by tobyMac
5. "Hold My Heart" by Tenth Avenue North
6. "When the Tears Fall" by Newsboys
7. "Learning to Breathe" by Switchfoot
8. "This Fragile Breath" by Todd Agnew
9. "It Is Well" by Kutless
10. "I'm Weak, You're Strong" by Mark Tedder
11. "Who Am I" by Casting Crowns
12. "Move (Keep Walkin')" by tobyMac
13. "Healing Begins" by Tenth Avenue North
14. "I'm Not Alright" by Sanctus Real
15. "Keep Fighting" by Fireflight
16. "Impossible" by Sidewalk Prophets
17. "Ready or Not" by Britt Nicole
18. "Praise You in This Storm" by Casting Crowns
19. "Strong Enough to Save" by Tenth Avenue North
20. "Cheer You On" by Jordan Feliz

ACKNOWLEDGMENTS

Special thanks to Chelsie, Jan, Sarah, Kathy R., Christina, Amanda, Melanie, Barbara, Chau, Lisa, Patty, Laura, Ian, Bethany, Kathy H., and everyone else who contributed to this book. I really appreciate you all opening up and discussing such personal subjects with me—I couldn't have done it without you!

Nikita Gill (*Your Soul is a River*), Rishika Sangreeta (https://www.facebook.com/r.s.poetry), Matt Eayre (*Reaching for the Light*), Nausicaa Twila (*Beautiful Minds Anonymous*), and the other poets whose work I quoted throughout the book: thank you for sharing such lovely words with me. I found them so encouraging, and I appreciate your gift.

I want to especially thank Janet Gugeler and Susan Sibley, who make the best editing team anyone could hope for. Thanks for taking the time, ladies!

I've been incredibly blessed with supportive coworkers, and I want everyone at work to know how much it means that you never doubt me when I tell you I'm having a tough pain day. You've been kind and patient with me, and for that I will be forever grateful.

Words seem inadequate to thank my family. Can we ever make people truly understand the way they touch our lives? I don't know. I do know that I would not be the person I am without my family. Without them…well, I'd have to write a whole 'nother book about how to get out of bed in the mornings, and the struggle would have nothing to do with having an invisible disability! I love you all so much, now and forever.

And speaking of words that are inadequate, I want to thank God for so much, so much of everything…not the least of which was His whisper in my ear, *"You should write a book about invisible disabilities."* Thanks for bringing me here.

ABOUT THE AUTHOR

Amy Anderson worked as a chef for seven years before her invisible disability caused her to pursue a writing career instead. She's worked with *The Sacrifice Anthology, Aelurus,* and *The Bird and Dog,* and is published in three separate *Chicken Soup for the Soul* books. You can reach her at contactamyanderson@gmail.com, follow her on Facebook at Shadow Lines Writing, or check out her blog at http://shadowlineswriting.tumblr.com/

[i] "McGill Pain Index," *RSDHope*
http://www.rsdhope.org/mcgill-pain-index---where-is-crps-pain-ranked.html
[ii] "Factsheet on Persons with Disabilities," *United Nations/WHO Enables: Development and Human Rights for All.* 2015.
http://www.un.org/disabilities/default.asp?id=18
[iii] "Americans With Disabilities Act," *United States Department of Justice Civil Rights Division*, 1990.
http://www.ada.gov/pubs/adastatute08.htm
[iv] "Americans With Disabilities Act," *United States Department of Justice Civil Rights Division*, 1990.
http://www.ada.gov/pubs/adastatute08.htm
[v] Cynthis K. Matthews, Nancy Grant Harrington, *Invisible disability*, (Mahwah, NJ: Lawrence Erlbaum Associates Publishers, 2000), 405-421.
[vi] "Disability Statistics: Facts & Statistics on Disabilities & Disability Issues," *Disabled World*, July 27, 2015.
http://www.disabled-world.com/disability/statistics/
[vii] "What is an Invisible Disability?" *Invisible Disabilities Association*, 2016. https://invisibledisabilities.org/what-is-an-invisible-disability/
[viii] "Don't Judge by Appearances." *Invisible Disabilities Association*, 2016. https://invisibledisabilities.org/ida-books-pamphlets/accessibleparking/dontjudgebyappearances/
[ix] Matthew 7:1-2, NLV
[x] Alecia M. Santuzzi, Pamela R. Waltz, Lisa M. Finkelstein, Deborah E. Rupp. "Invisible Disabilities: Unique Challenges for Employees and Organizations." *Industrial and Organizational Psychology* 7, 2. April 22, 2014, 204-219
[xi] "Factsheet on Persons with Disabilities," *United Nations/WHO Enables: Development and Human Rights for All.* 2015.
http://www.un.org/disabilities/default.asp?id=18
[xii] Disability Statistics: Facts & Statistics on Disabilities & Disability Issues," *Disabled World*, July 27, 2015.
http://www.disabled-world.com/disability/statistics/
[xiii] "Don't Judge by Appearances." *Invisible Disabilities Association*, 2016. https://invisibledisabilities.org/ida-books-pamphlets/accessibleparking/dontjudgebyappearances/
[xiv] "Don't Judge by Appearances." *Invisible Disabilities Association*, 2016. https://invisibledisabilities.org/ida-books-

pamphlets/accessibleparking/dontjudgebyappearances/

[xv] Allen Appel, "Invisible disabilities come in many forms," *TC Palm,* February 17, 2008.
http://www.tcpalm.com/lifestyle/allan-appel-invisible-disabilities-come-in-many-forms-ep-404323103-338755081.html

[xvi] Mary Yerkes, "When We Suffer: A Biblical Perspective on Chronic Pain and Illness." *Focus on the Family*, 2007.
http://www.focusonthefamily.com/lifechallenges/emotional-health/living-with-chronic-pain-and-illness/when-we-suffer-a-biblical-perspective-on-chronic-pain-and-illness

[xvii] Mary Yerkes. "Remaining Positive When Facing a Chronic Illness," *Focus on the Family*, 2007.
http://www.focusonthefamily.com/lifechallenges/emotional-health/living-with-chronic-pain-and-illness/remaining-positive-when-facing-a-chronic-illness

[xviii] Georgia Shaffer, *A Gift of Mourning Glories—Restoring Your Life After Loss* (Servant Publications, 2000).